THE DR. BARBARA NATURAL HEALING COOKBOOK

PLANT BASED DIET

BY

KATHY D. THURMAN

Disclaimer

This book contains material that is intended solely for informative purposes. For medical advice, please see your healthcare practitioner. In particular, the author disclaims any liability arising from the use or use of this book's contents.

Table of Contents

INTRODUCTION

HERBAL ALKALINE DIET OF DR. BARBARA

Unfortunately, a lot of the stuff we eat nowadays is acidic meat, dairy, sugar, etc. The average Western diet of today is heavy in processed, genetically modified, and hybridized foods, which throw off the blood's alkalinity balance.

Dr. Barbara recommended sticking to natural meals created by God and avoiding all other foods. The foundation of Dr. Barbara's therapeutic approach is the notion that sickness can only live in an acidic environment. Thus, "alkalize the environment and get rid of the disease" became his mantra. It is well known that the body works continuously to keep the blood's pH level at a healthy 7.4. If we eat an electric diet that is naturally alkaline based, we may assist it in achieving and maintaining this equilibrium.

Unfortunately, there are a lot of very acidic items in the average Western diet. It lacks nutrients yet is delicious and convenient. The foundation of Dr. Barbara's regimen is the notion that the Western diet's lack of nourishment stems from its heavy processing. For this reason, he insisted on eating meals rich in more than 100 minerals, which promote the body's general vigor and electrical activity.

CHAPTER 1

PRINCIPLES OF DR. BARBARA DIETS

- Only items on the Dr. Barbara Food List are permitted to be consumed.

You should only consume the items on Dr. Barbara's list of permitted foods, he stressed.

All-natural alkaline foods are included in the list, even though it is very limited and leaves out a lot of items. Furthermore, Dr. Barbara emphasized that consuming any modified food is not advised. He meant all plants generated by artificial cross-pollination are hybridized meals. The majority of fruits and vegetables in the market today are hybridized.

Even though the Dr. Barbara diet appears to be somewhat limited, you may still use the permitted ingredients to make delicious, nutritious, and well-balanced meals. The fact that so much of the food we consume today is hybridized is one of the reasons so many items have been left off the list. According to Dr. Barbara, hybridized fruits and vegetables typically have a reduced nutritional content and are artificial, not electric. A plant can be identified as hybridized if it lacks seeds, for example. These days, there are a lot of fruit options available without seeds, such as watermelon, oranges, grapes, tomatoes, berries, etc. Ignore these at all costs. Natural foods, in Dr. Barbara's opinion, are far healthier than foods produced by humans.

CHAPTER 2

IMPORTANT KITCHEN UTILITIES

Cooking is like most other activities in that it requires specific instruments. Essential kitchen appliances can be divided into groups based on their intended uses.

- Silverware

Spoons, knives, forks, ladles, spatulas, tongs, slotted spoons, whisks, and so forth are among them.

- Cutting implements

This category includes everything that is used for chopping, slicing, crushing, or grinding, such as graters, potato mashers, vegetable peelers, knives, etc.

- Storage containers secure from ovens

Nothing is easier than putting your meal prep containers directly into the oven after removing them from the refrigerator. If your items will need to be reheated differently, try to keep them in various containers. For instance, a container of roasted chicken would go in the toaster oven, while a container of wild rice or quinoa would go right into a steamer.

- A slow cooker

An excellent tool for reheating prepared meals or for lunch.

- A Strong Blender
- A Juicer Food Processor
- An oven toaster
- A kettle for tea
- Pots & Pans

These appliances such as a spiralizer, air fryer, instant cooker, sandwich maker, steamer basket, zester for key limes, etc. may be useful, but you can live without them.

- Other

Can openers, corkscrews, measuring cups and spoons, pepper mills, salad spinners, colanders and strainers, chopping boards, pots and pans, mixing bowls, and other unclassified objects are common in most kitchens?

Cutlery, pots and pans, and other kitchen essentials are among the items that every kitchen should have. The rest, you should obtain if you can, but you don't have to strive to obtain them all at once. You can purchase one or two items from each category to begin with, and then progressively add more if you feel like you need them. If you are unable to obtain the majority of these items, remember that our ancestors cooked delicious meals with a meager supply of cooking utensils and sometimes without power.

Furthermore, the kitchen utensils you require rely not only on your spending limit but also on the kinds of meals you want to cook. For instance, you will want kitchen scales if you frequently bake, a blender if smoothies are a regular component of your diet, etc.

CHAPTER 3

NUTRITIONAL STEP-BY-STEP GUIDE BY DR. BARBARA

Since the body can create all the acid it needs, high urine pH levels indicate that the body is attempting to get rid of extra acid. Acidic meals and drinks allow this extra acid to enter your organs.

Luckily, your body works hard to keep things balanced and eliminates excess acid because it cannot stand it. But if you consistently eat a lot of acidic food over months or years, your kidneys and lungs will eventually be unable to handle the excess, and you might end up with acidosis. The majority of the excess acids are derived from proteins. For this reason, Dr. Barbara had little interest in proteins and amino acids. If you can't avoid or minimize protein, there's a straightforward fix for this issue: consume more alkaline foods (fruits and vegetables). Alkaline meals will lower acid levels in this way. The issue is that too many neutral foods, such as sweets, fats, and carbohydrates, are present in the modern diet and cannot balance out an excess of acidity.

If you wish to enjoy the health advantages of an alkaline lifestyle, your diet should mostly consist of the foods on Dr. Barbara's food list. Even though you might not be able to get many of the foods on this list where you live, it's still simple to make delicious and interesting dinners with only a few of the items.

Dr. BARBARA SALAD RECIPES

ALKALINE SALADS AND SALAD BURRITOS

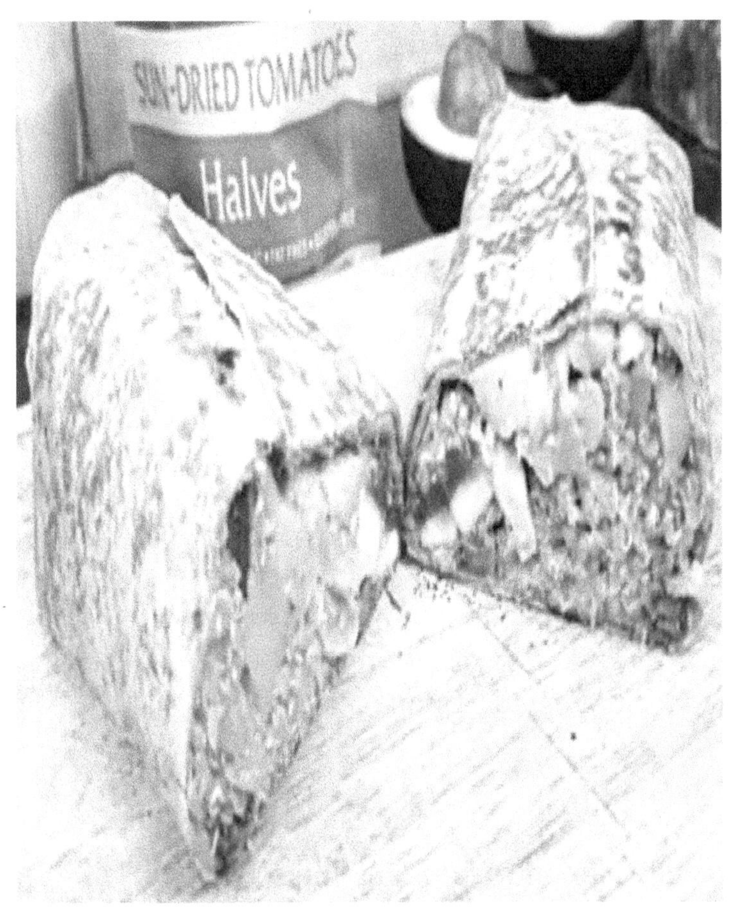

Neither meat nor potatoes are present. It is a substitute for hamburgers. Consume food to get health and energy. Try your hand at it. You will adore it.

Servings: Two

Time spent preparing: ten minutes; cooking: five minutes;

Information about nutrition: 29 g Carb; 4.4 g Fiber; 9.1 g Fats; 11.5 g Protein; 274 Cal

Components

Arugula, 2 ounces; ¼ cup cherry tomatoes

Two teaspoons of homemade tahini butter

Half a cup of cooked lentils

Two tortillas made using Kamut flour

Bonus:

One tablespoon of key lime juice

One-half teaspoon each of salt and cayenne pepper

Guidelines

1. To make the dressing, take a small bowl, add the tahini butter, and toss in the lime juice until well combined.

2. Transfer the tomatoes to a medium-sized bowl, add the arugula and chickpeas, pour in the dressing, toss to combine, cover the bowl, and refrigerate for 20 minutes.

3. Just before serving, reheat the tortillas, stuff them with the chickpea mixture, season with cayenne and salt, and roll them up.

THE MANGO SALAD WITH RAINBOW COLORS

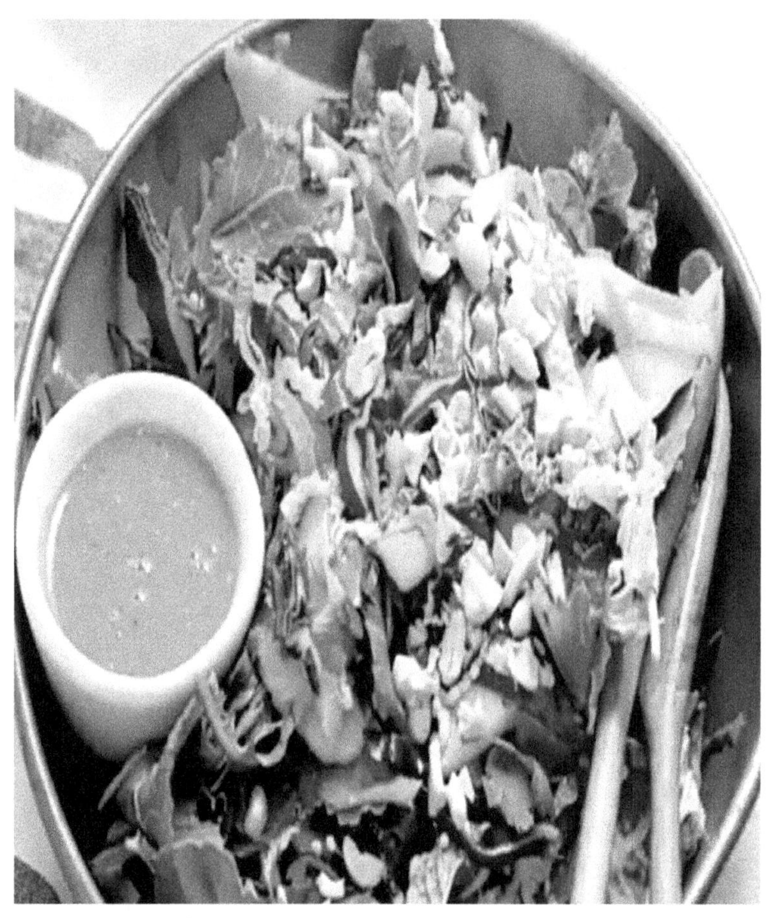

Cook this when you're feeling particularly spiritual, when you need a comforting meal, or when you have a cold (though vegans don't typically get cold).

Get ready for this, and when you take it down, you'll feel like a global conqueror.

Servings: Two

Ten minutes for preparation; no time for cooking;

108 calories, 0.5 grams of fat, 1 gram of protein, 28.1 grams of carbohydrates, and 3.3 grams of fiber.

Components

One peeled, destoned, cubed mango; one chopped onion; one chopped cup cherry tomatoes; one split cucumber; one sliced, deseeded green bell pepper

Additional: 1/3 tsp salt

One-half teaspoon of cayenne

half a key lime, squeezed

Guidelines

1. Fill a medium-sized bowl with the mango chunks, onion, tomatoes, bell pepper, and cucumber. Drizzle with lime juice.

2. Add cayenne pepper and salt, mix to blend, and let the salad sit in the fridge for at least 20 minutes.

3. Present immediately.

THE PLEASANT SPRING SALAD

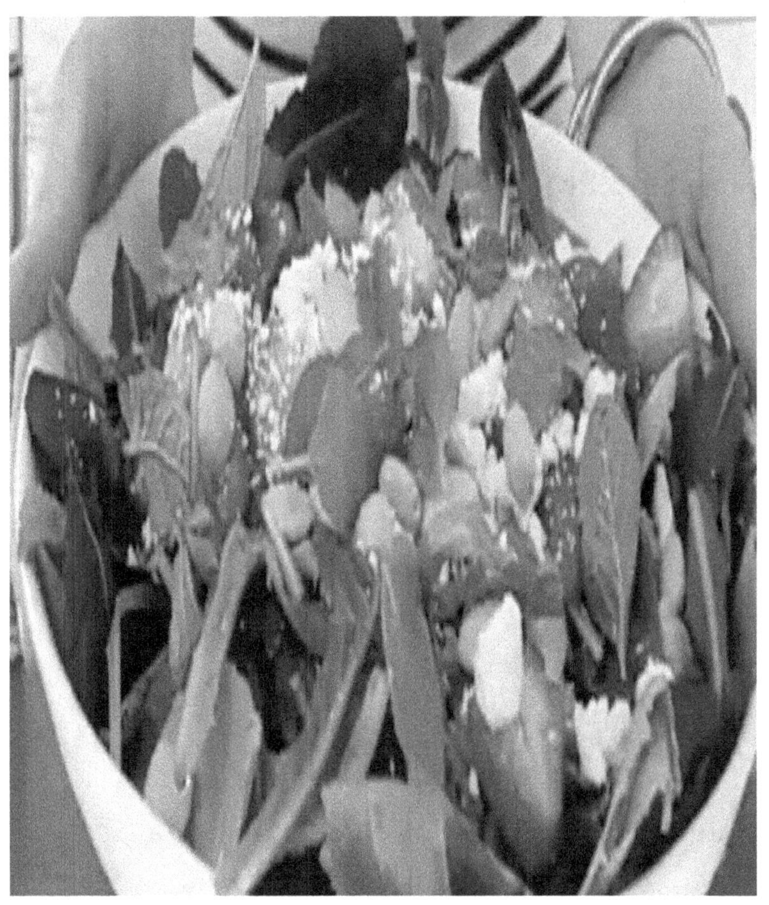

Perhaps you don't reside in the Caribbean or Mediterranean region. You can still eat this, it's alright. Do it in a corner, please. I'm joking. Wasn't it delicious?

Servings: Two

It takes five minutes to prepare and ten minutes to cook.

Information about nutrition: 87.3 kcal; 1.3 g Fiber; 6 g Carb; 1.4 g Protein; 7 g Fats;

Components

Four ounces of arugula

Half a cup of cherry tomatoes and a half cup of basil leaves

Juiced half a key lime

Two teaspoons of walnuts

Additional: ¼ tsp salt

one-eighth teaspoon of cayenne

One-third cup tahini butter

Guidelines

1. To make the dressing, take a small bowl, fill it with key lime juice, then add the tahini butter, cayenne pepper, and salt. Whisk everything together.

2. Transfer the arugula, tomatoes, and basil leaves to a medium-sized bowl, add the dressing, and use your hands to massage.

3. After letting the salad sit for 20 minutes, taste it and adjust the seasoning before serving.

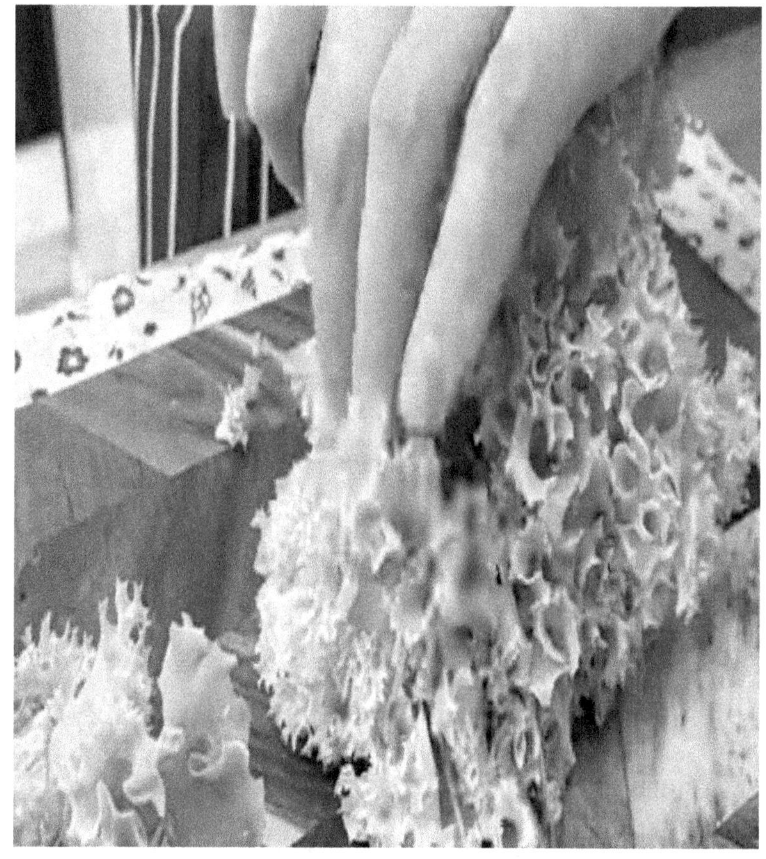

"You will reap deliciousness from the electric greens you sow." Yes, indeed.

Okay, so this salad tastes really good I mean, really good rather than simply being "green."

Servings: Two

Time spent preparing: five minutes; time spent cooking: none;

Information about nutrition: 12.5 g Fats, 1.6 g Protein, 7.8 g Carb, 1 g Fiber, and 142 Cal

Components

one-half cucumber, seeded

Four ounces of arugula

one-eighth teaspoon of salt

One tablespoon of key lime juice

One tablespoon of olive oil

one-eighth teaspoon of cayenne

Guidelines

1. Slice the cucumber and place it in a salad dish with the arugula.

2. Pour the oil and lime juice mixture over the salad, stir to mix, and add cayenne and salt to taste.

3. After tossing to combine, serve.

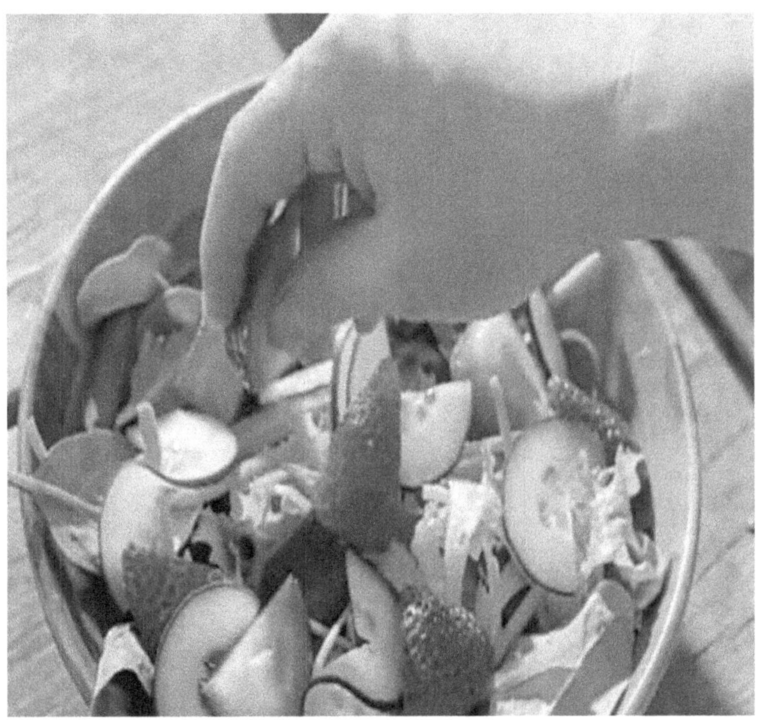

It's always a good idea to use dandelions. Superfood with a ton of nutrients.

You've got a winner when you combine the tastes of berries with onion. Have fun!

Servings: Two

It takes ten minutes to prepare and seven minutes to cook.

204 calories, 16.1 grams of fat, 7 grams of protein, 10.6 grams of carbohydrates, and 2.8 grams of fiber.

Components

half an onion, peeled and sliced; five strawberries; two cups of dandelion greens, cut and washed;

One tablespoon of key lime juice

One tablespoon of oil made from grapeseed

Additional: ¼ tsp salt

Guidelines

1. Heat a medium-sized skillet pans over medium heat, add oil, and let it warm up.

2. Add onion, stir to combine, season with 1/8 teaspoon salt, and sauté for 3 to 5 minutes, or until soft and golden brown.

3. In the meantime, put the strawberry slices in a small bowl, pour in ½ tablespoon of lime juice, and toss to coat.

4. After the onions are golden brown, add the remaining lime juice, swirl to combine, and cook for one minute more.

5. Take the pan off of the burner, put the onions in a big salad bowl, add the strawberries and their juices, the dandelion greens, and finally sprinkle with the remaining salt. After tossing until combined, serve.

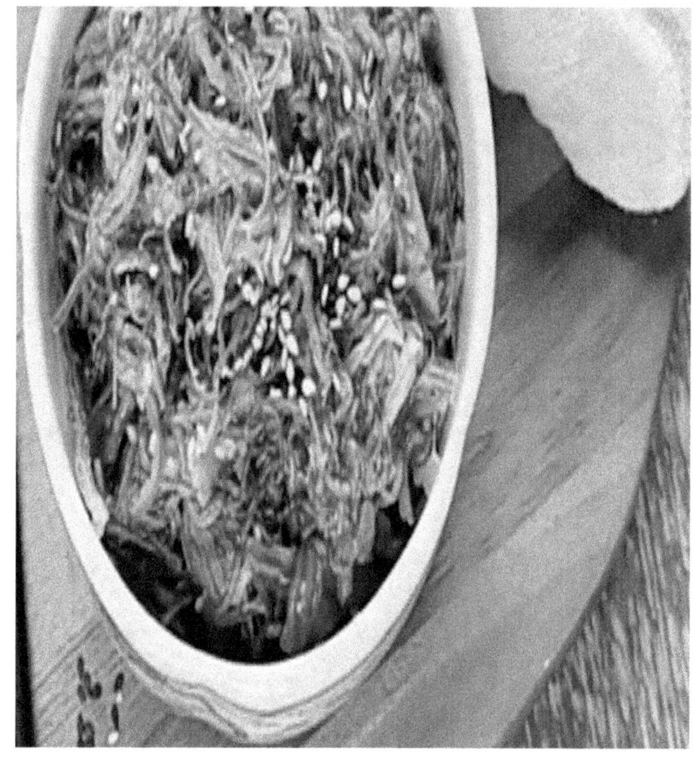

The wakame stems shouldn't alarm you; they're not only well-integrated but also healthful. Savor this flavorful meal on a sunny, bright day. Enjoy your meal!

Servings: Two

Take fifteen minutes to prepare; No cooking time is required.

Information about nutrition: 3.6 g Fats, 3 g Protein, 8 g Carb, 1.7 g Fiber; 106 Cal

Components

One cup of wakame stems

One-third cup finely chopped red bell pepper

One-half teaspoon of onion powder

1/4 cup key lime juice

Bonus:

A quarter-tsp agave syrup

One-third cup of sesame seeds

One-third cup of sesame oil

Guidelines

1. Put the stems of the wakame in a basin, fill it with water, and let it soak for ten minutes before draining.

2. In the meantime, make the dressing. To do this, put the onion, lime juice, agave syrup, and sesame oil in a small bowl and whisk to combine.

3. Fill a big plate with the drained wakame stems, add the bell pepper, drizzle with the dressing, and toss to coat.

4. Top the salad with sesame seeds and serve.

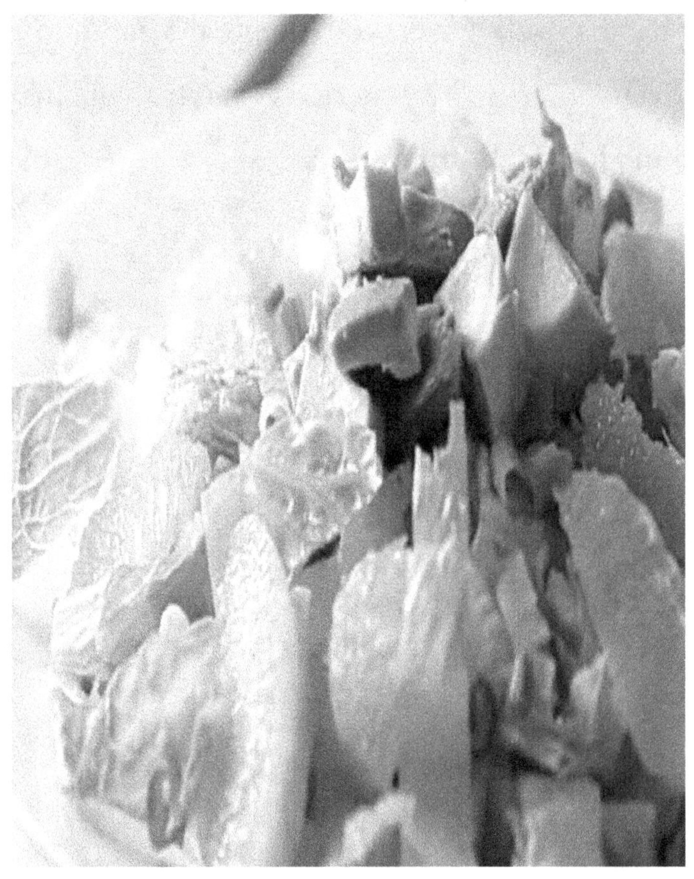

Do you want to laugh out loud? Pronounce the name of this dish loudly.

Alright, so maybe it wasn't hilarious, but this is tasty and easy to carry in addition to being healthful. The dressing is stuck in the bottom of the greens-filled jar. Brilliant! Yes, I am aware. It also blends well when you dump the jar into a bowl. Or, after a few vigorous shakes, you may consume it straight from the jar.

Servings: Two

Time spent preparing: five minutes; time spent cooking: none;

Information about nutrition: 14.7 g Carb; 7 g Fiber; 18.9 g Fats; 3.3 g Protein; 228 Cal;

Components

One peeled and sliced orange

four cups of greens

Half an avocado, pitted, chopped, and peeled

Two teaspoons of red onion, slivered

1/4 cup of cilantro

Additional: ¼ tsp salt

Half a cup of olive oil

Lime juice, two teaspoons

two tsp orange juice

Guidelines

1. To make the dressing, put the cilantro in a food processor with the oil, lime juice, orange juice, and salt. Pulse to mix.

2. Transfer the salad dressing to a mason jar. Toss with remaining ingredients and transfer to a salad dish or serve in a jar.

THE SUCCULENT ELECTRICAL SALAD

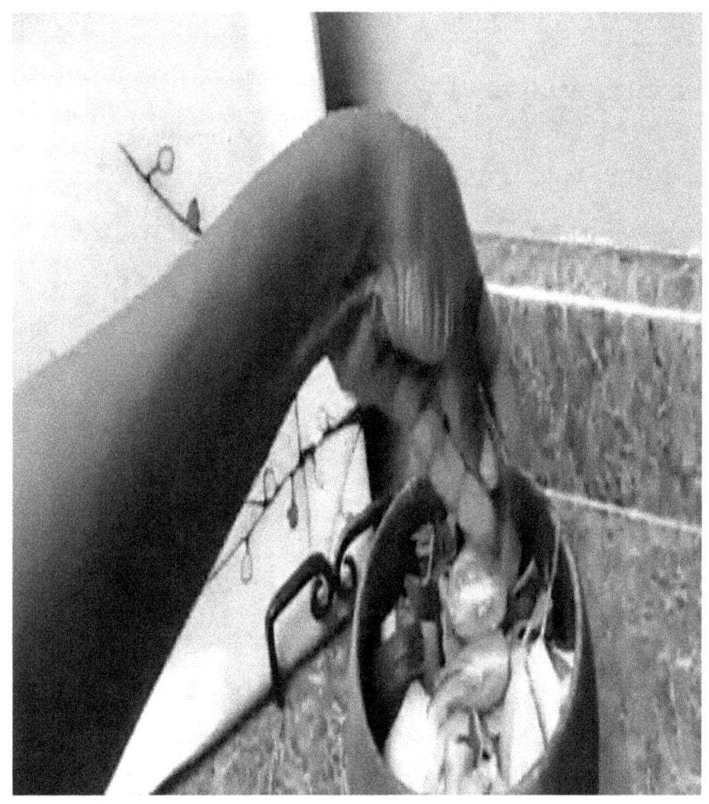

Serves two people. That's it. However, refrain from touching your neighbor's mason jar salad. Come on, this vegan salad is alkaline and healthful.

Servings: Two

The preparation took five minutes. No cooking time is required.

129 calories, 7 grams of fat, 2 grams of protein, 14 grams of carbohydrates, and 4 grams of fiber.

Components

one-third of a medium cucumber, peeled and diced; six lettuce leaves, broken into pieces

Chop six cherry tomatoes, four mushrooms, and ten olives

Bonus: ½ lime, juiced

One tsp olive oil

One-half teaspoon of salt

Guidelines

1. Transfer all the ingredients to a medium-sized salad bowl and toss to combine.

2. Present immediately.

THE SUPERFOOD SALAD WITH FONIO

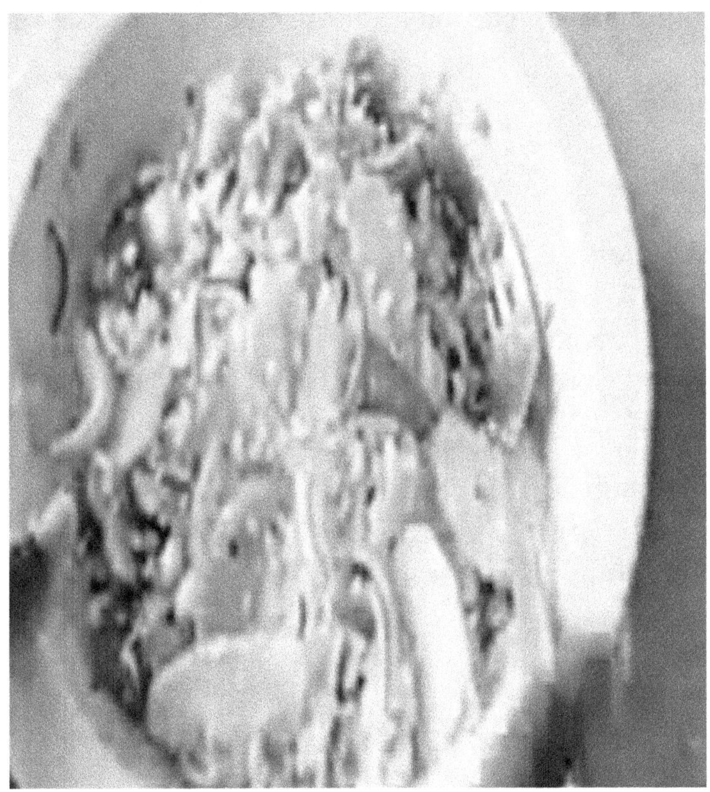

Servings: Two

Time spent preparing: ten minutes; cooking: five minutes;

145 calories, 3 grams of fat, 6 grams of protein, 24.5 grams of carbohydrates, and 5.5 grams of fiber.

Components

1/4 cup cooked lentils and 1/4 cup finely sliced cucumber

½ cup finely diced red pepper

Half a cup of cherry tomatoes

half a cup of Fonio

one-third teaspoon of salt

One spoonful of oil made from grapeseed

one-eighth teaspoon of cayenne

One key lime squeezed

a single cup of spring water

Guidelines

1. Fill a medium pot with water, set it on high heat, and bring it to a boil.

2. Add the Fonio, reduce the heat to low, cook for one minute, and then take the pan off of the burner.

3. Put the pan's cover on, let the Fonio rest for five minutes, then fluff it with a fork and allow it to cool for fifteen minutes.

4. In a salad bowl, mix the oil and lime juice. Next, add the salt and cayenne pepper.

5. Include the Fonio and add the remaining ingredients. Toss to combine, and serve.

THE HEALTHY SALAD OF CHICKPEA ROAST

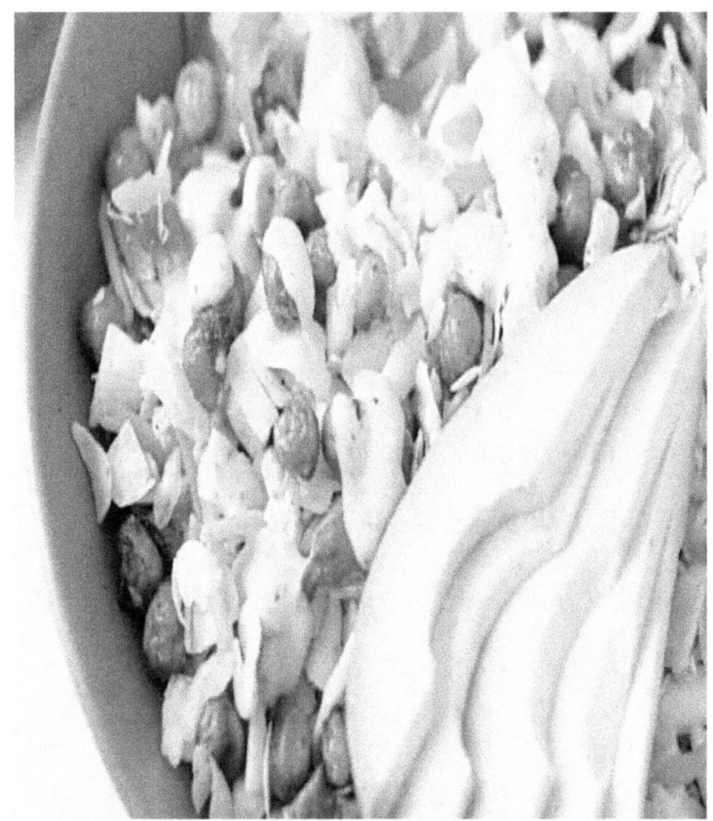

Servings: Two

It takes ten minutes to prepare and twenty minutes to cook.

Information about nutrition: 208.3 calories; 30 g of carbohydrates; 8 g of fats; 6.4 g of protein;

Components

½ cup of sliced, deseeded cucumber

Two avocados, diced, pitted and peeled

One medium white onion, chopped and peeled

two cups of boiled lentils

¼ cup finely chopped coriander

Bonus:

One tsp powdered onion

One-half teaspoon of cayenne

One-teaspoonful Sea salt

Two teaspoons of shelled hemp seeds

One key lime squeezed

One tablespoon of olive oil

Guidelines

1. Turn on the oven, then warm it to 425 degrees Fahrenheit.

In the meantime, spread some oil on a baking sheet, add some salt, pepper, and onion powder to the chickpeas, and toss to incorporate.

3. After the chickpeas have baked for 20 minutes, or until they are crisp and golden brown, allow them to cool for 10 minutes.

4. Move the chickpeas into a basin, then incorporate the additional ingredients by stirring them well. Serve immediately.

THE SALAD TAMABOULEH (AMARANTHA)

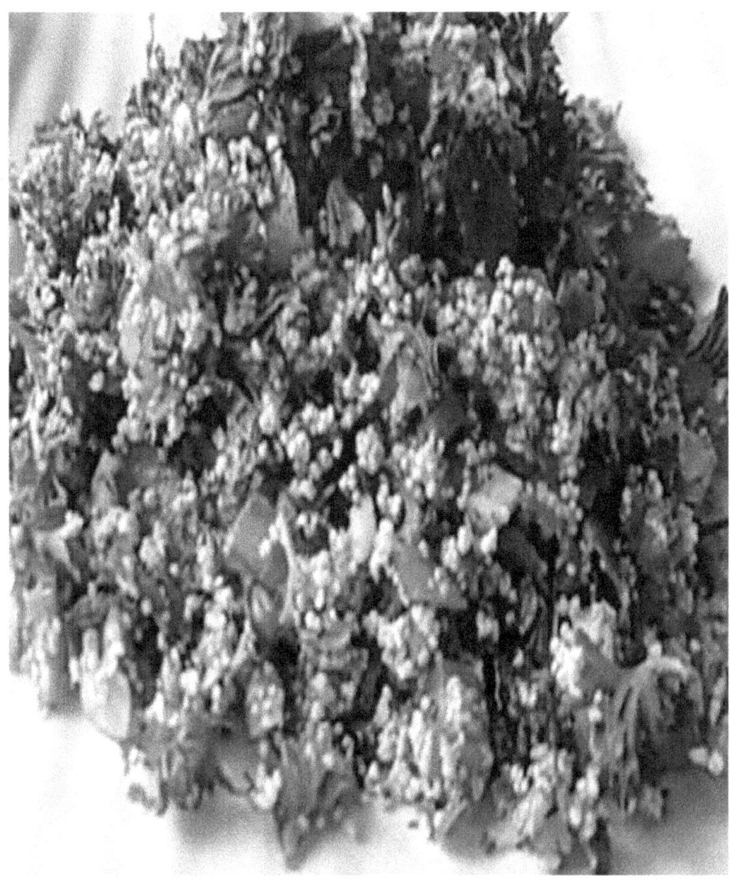

It's time to devour this salad now! We're going to serve you a meal so rich it will make your eyes water.

Servings: Two

It takes five minutes to prepare and ten minutes to cook.

Information about nutrition: 214 calories, 37 g carbs, 4.5 g fats, 6.5 g protein, and 9 g fiber;

Components

one little white onion, sliced and peeled

One cup of prepared amaranth

½ cup chopped, deseeded cucumber

One cup of cooked lentils

½ chopped medium red bell pepper

Additional: 1/3 tsp sea salt

one-eighth teaspoon of cayenne

Key lime juice, two teaspoons

Guidelines

1. Fill a small bowl with lime juice, then add salt and swirl to mix.

2. Transfer the remaining components to a salad dish, pour in the lime juice combination, toss to combine, and serve.

THE DR. BARBARA ZUCCHINI AND THE BOWL OF MUSHROOMS

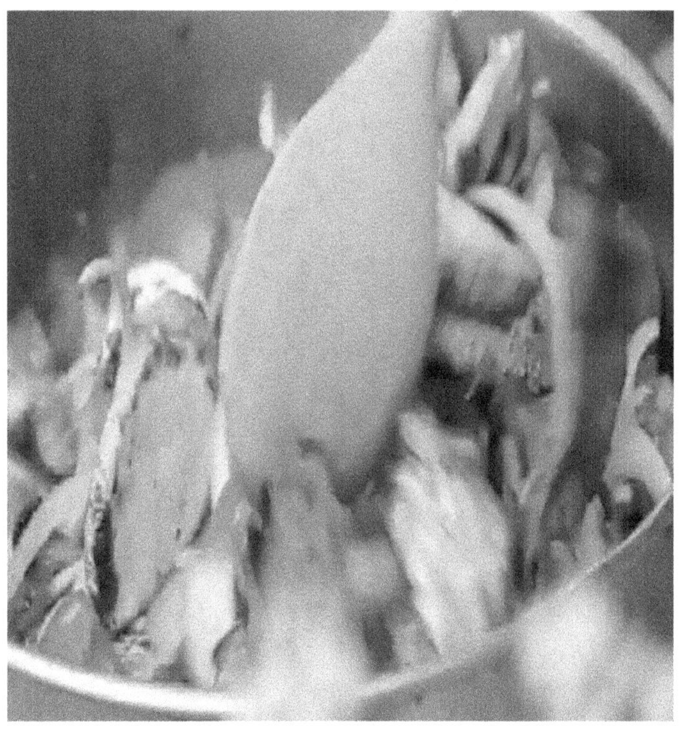

One of the first vegan recipes I ever learned was this one, which I changed and named after my mentor, Dr. Barbara. I detested zucchini and didn't think plants could be prepared to taste as meaty and umami-like as vegetables, but this blew my head. Though after this you won't think the same. I promise it.

Servings: Two

It takes five minutes to prepare and eight minutes to cook.

Information about nutrition: 2 g Fats, 0.9 g Protein, 36 g Carb, and 6 g Fiber; 168 Cal

Components

Two spiralized zucchini

½ cup sliced mushrooms; ½ of medium red bell pepper, sliced

½ sliced medium green bell pepper ½ sliced peeled medium white onion

Additional: 1/3 tsp salt

one-eighth teaspoon of cayenne

One spoonful of oil made from grapeseed

Guidelines

1. Heat a large frying pan over medium-high heat. Add oil. When the pan is heated, add the onion, bell peppers, and mushrooms. Cook for three to five minutes, or until the vegetables are crisp-tender.

2. Include the zucchini noodles, stir to combine, and heat for an additional two minutes.

3. Present immediately.

ALKALINE PEAR CRÈME

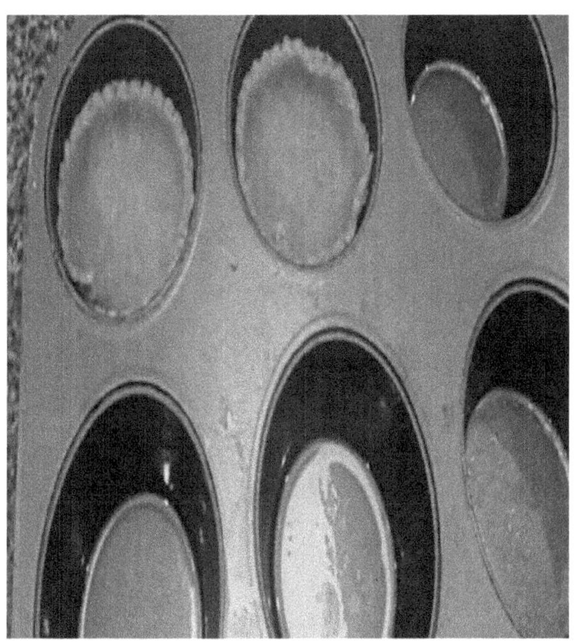

Servings: Two

It will take ten minutes to prepare and fifteen minutes to cook.

Information about nutrition: 76.1 kcal; 14.3 g carbs; 0.9 g fiber; 3.3 g fats; 0.9 g protein;

Components

1/3 cup of spelt flour

a half-cup of finely chopped peach

One tsp finely chopped burro banana

2.3 tsp finely chopped walnuts

6 ½ teaspoons homemade walnut milk

Bonus:

a one-sixteenth teaspoon of salt

Two and a third tablespoons of date sugar

1/3 spoonful of heated spring water

two and a third teaspoon of key lime juice

Guidelines

1. Turn on the oven, then warm it to 400 degrees Fahrenheit.

2. In the meantime, peel, split in half, remove the pit, and chop one half into ½-inch pieces, setting aside the other half for later use.

3. Transfer the milk into a medium-sized bowl, and then thoroughly mix in the mashed burro banana and lime juice.

4. Transfer the flour to a different medium bowl, toss in the date sugar, and salt, whisk in the milk mixture until smooth, then fold in the peaches until incorporated.

5. Grease four silicone muffin tins with oil, pour the prepared batter into each one evenly, and top with walnuts.

6. Bake the muffins for ten to fifteen minutes, or until the toothpick put into each muffin comes out clean and the tops are pleasantly golden brown.

7. After muffins are done, let them cool for ten minutes before serving.

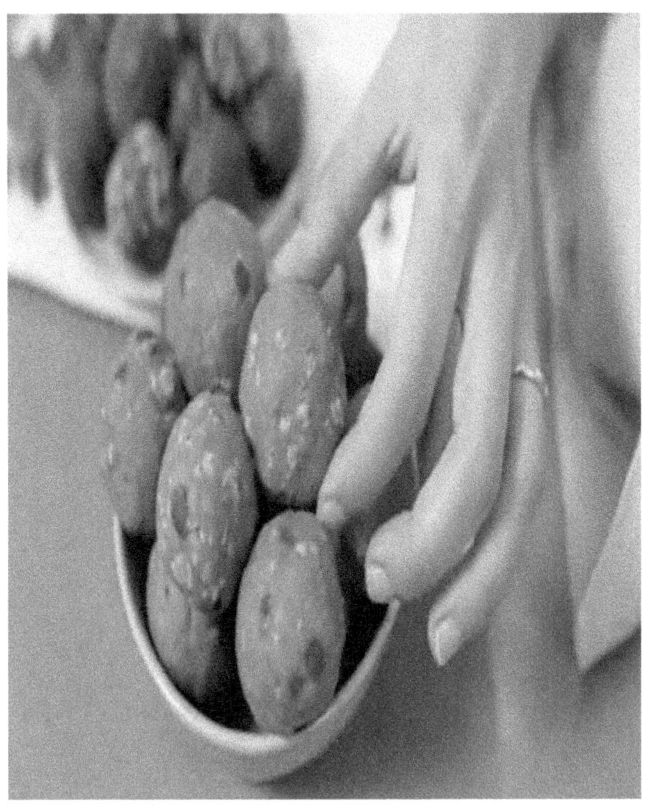

Since eggs are needed for Matzo balls, this recipe requires some creativity. Fortunately, we were able to crack the code and avoid breaking any eggs. Better still, there's a ton of protein in this meal!

feeds one hungry person for two meals or two hungry persons for one meal. Have fun!

Servings: Two

Ten minutes for preparation; no time for cooking;

Information about nutrition: 8 g Fats, 2 g Protein, 10 g Carb, 1 g Fiber, and 119 Cal

Components

Half a cup of blueberries

Half a cup of dehydrated dates

One cup of shredded soft-jelly coconut

Half a cup of walnuts

One-half teaspoon of date sugar

Additional: ½ tsp agave syrup

a one-sixteenth teaspoon of salt.

Guidelines

1. Put the walnuts in a food processor and pulse the mixture until a fine powder is achieved.

2. Next, pulse in the dates, coconut, berries, and date sugar until well combined. Next, gradually blend in the agave syrup until the soft paste comes together.

3. Transfer the mixture to a medium-sized dish, let it cool for at least half an hour, and then portion the mixture into balls, using one tablespoon of the mixture for each ball.

4. After rolling the balls in additional coconut, serve.

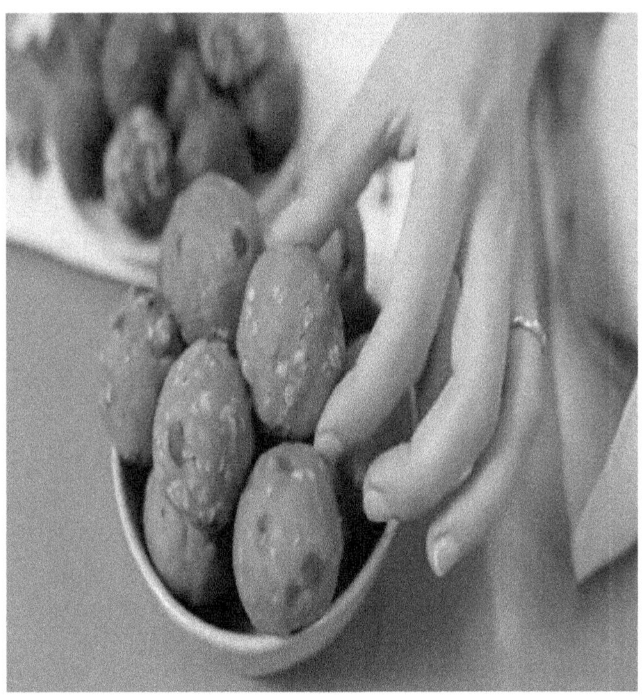

In Los Angeles, people prefer to believe that males are to blame for everyone's

inability to settle down. Given that Peter Pan, a legendary figure from Disney, is always in flight, the name makes sense. You won't want to settle down after receiving the power and energy these energy balls will provide you.

Servings: Two

The preparation took five minutes. No cooking time is required.

Information about nutrition: 8 g Fats, 1 g Protein, 11 g Carb, 2 g Fiber, 123 Cal

Components

1/4 cup raspberries

Five occasions

1/16 teaspoon of sea salt

one-third cup of walnuts

1 ½ cups shredded soft-jelly coconut

Guidelines

1. Fill the jar of a high-speed food processor or blender with all the ingredients.

2. After placing the lid on the blender jar, pulse for 40 to 60 seconds, or until everything is fully blended.

3. Using your moist hands, form the dough into balls, using one tablespoon of the mixture for each ball. Put the balls on the tray and freeze for at least thirty minutes.

4. Serve immediately.

THE BAKED ZUCCHINI PANCAKES

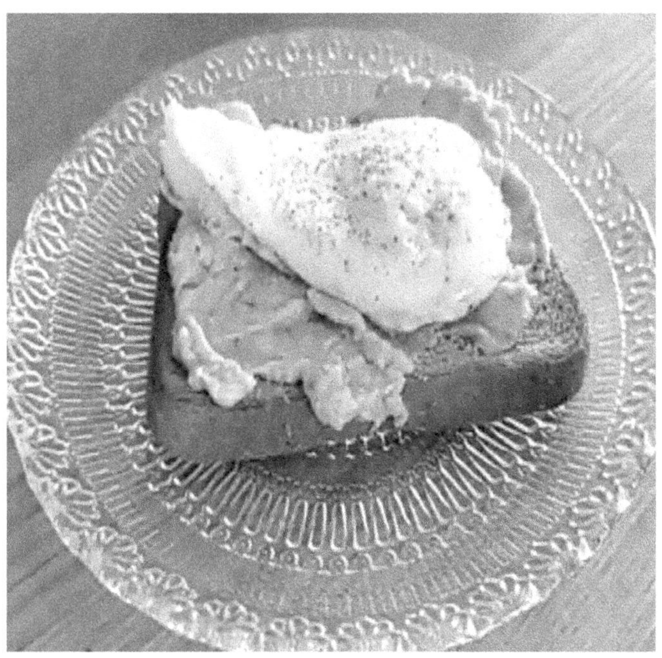

I am aware that the health community has a negative opinion of pancakes. However, what exactly makes it awful? ingredients, naturally! If every component was healthy, I'll wager that it would also be healthy! However, the ingredients in this recipe make them healthful and fantastic.

Servings: Two

Time spent preparing: 10 minutes; Cooking period: eight minutes.

Information about nutrition: 130 calories, 4 g fats, 3 g protein, 21 g carbs, and 3 g fiber;

Components

One cup of spelt flour

½ cup chopped walnuts and ½ cup grated zucchini

One cup of homemade walnut milk

Bonus:

One spoonful of sugar with dates

One spoonful of oil made from grapeseed

Guidelines

1. In a medium-sized bowl, combine the flour and date sugar; swirl to combine.

2. Pour milk and mashed burro banana into it, whisking until smooth batter forms. Fold in zucchini and almonds just until combined.

3. Heat a sizable frying pan over medium-high heat. Add oil to the pan. Once heated, divide the batter into portions and form each part into a pancake.

4. Cook for three to four minutes on each side before serving each pancake.

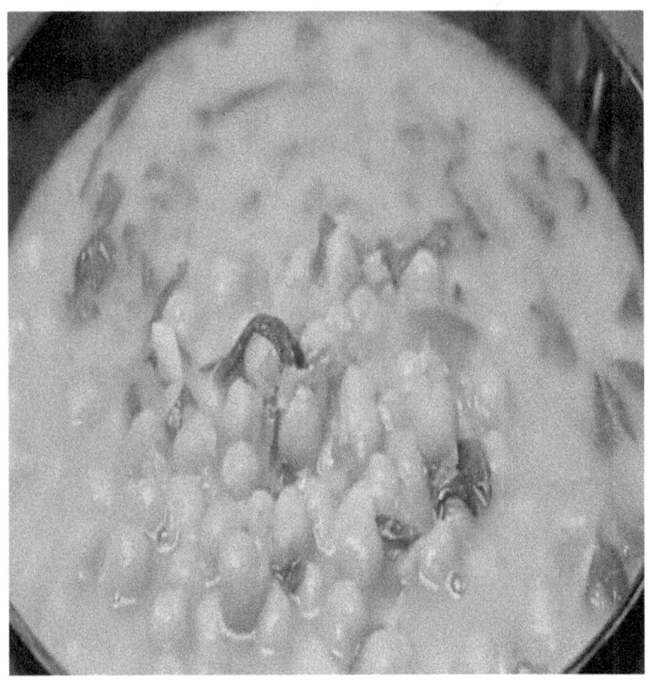

For those of you who are familiar with chicken nuggets, you are aware of its popularity. Hey, this isn't Chicken, though. We decided to give this recipe a try and transform it into the ideal fish or chicken substitute. Have fun!

Servings: Two

Time spent preparing: 10 minutes; cooking: 30 minutes;

Information about nutrition: 291.6 calories, 3.9 g fats, 19.9 g protein, 26.8 g carbohydrates, and 3.4 g fiber;

Components

two cups of boiled lentils

Half a teaspoon of salt

One tsp powdered onion

1 tablespoon and 1/3 cup of bread crumbs

Guidelines

1. Turn on the oven, then warm it to 350 degrees Fahrenheit.

2. In the meantime, pulse the chickpeas in a food processor until they become crumbly.

Place the chickpeas into a bowl, add all the other ingredients (except the 1/3 cup of breadcrumbs), and stir until a thick mixture forms.

4. Form the dough into uniformly sized balls, then roll each ball into a nugget. Place the balls on an oil-greased baking sheet and bake for 15 minutes on each side or until golden brown.

5. Present immediately.

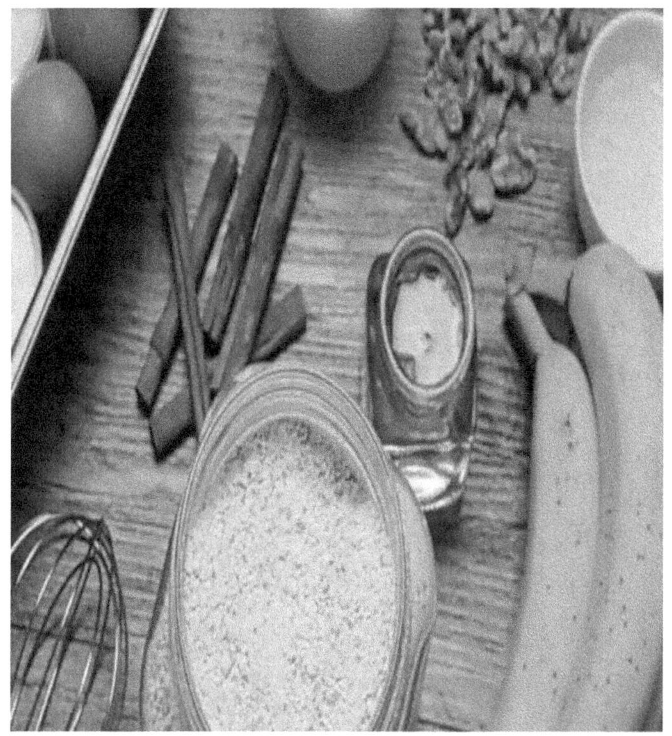

This doesn't need to be explained. Make it happen.

Thank you very much.

Servings: Two

It takes ten minutes to prepare and twenty minutes to cook.

Nutrition information: 186 calories, 2 g fiber, 1.3 g protein, 11.3 g fat, and 22 g carbs.

Components

1/3 cup chopped walnuts

1 1/3 cup of burro banana

1/3 cup of spelt flour

1/8 teaspoon salt ¼ cup agave syrup

Extra: 1 1/3 teaspoons olive oil

Guidelines

1. Switch on the oven, then set it to 350 degrees F and let it preheat.

2. In the meantime, put the burro banana in a medium-sized bowl, mash it with a fork, and then stir in the agave syrup and oil until well combined.

3. Transfer the flour to a different medium bowl, add the nuts and salt, and whisk to combine. Next, add the burro banana mixture and stir until smooth.

4. Transfer the mixture into a loaf pan lined with parchment paper, and bake for 20 minutes, or until the top becomes golden brown and the cake is firm.

5. After the bread is finished, let it cool for ten minutes before slicing it and serving.

THE PUDDING SEA MOSS INVIGORATING

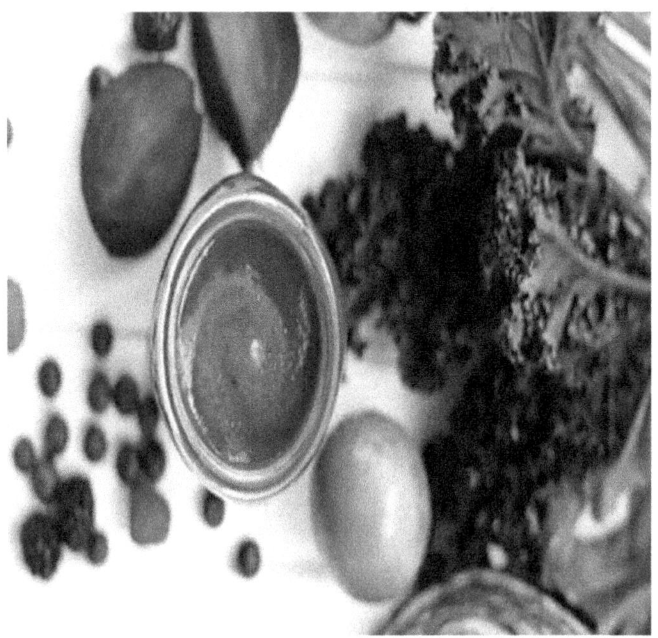

Whether you're heading up a mountain or running a board meeting, this delectable pudding will set you up for success. It's packed with iron, vitamins, and minerals that will keep your body and mind well-fed.

Servings: Two

The preparation took five minutes. No cooking time is required.

Information about nutrition: 0.7 g Protein, 0.5 g Fats, 23.4 g Carb, and 2.8 g Fiber; 97.8 Cal

Components

2 peeled burro bananas

Two cups of blueberries

Half a cup of sea moss gel

A quarter-cup of spring Directions for Water

1. Attach the jar to a high-speed food processor or blender, then pour all ingredients aside from water into it.

2. Put the lid on the blender jar, pulse it until smooth, and then gradually mix in water until the desired thickness is reached.

3. Present immediately.

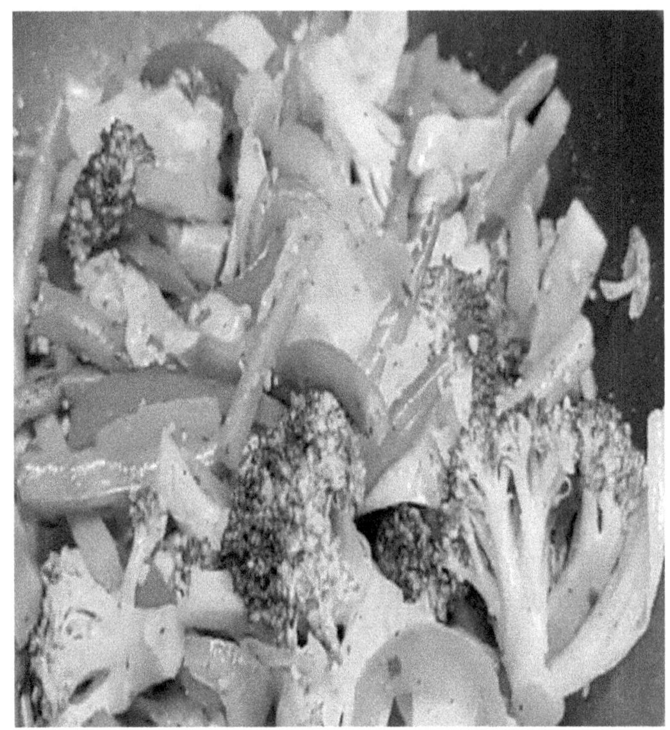

Growing up, this was one of my favorite meals. Since I no longer eat eggs, it was time to replicate the hearty dish using mashed avocado.

Servings: Two

The preparation took five minutes. No cooking time is required.

Information about nutrition: 189 Cal; 20 g Carb; 5.4 g Fiber; 11 g Fats; 3 g Protein;

Components

Two toasted spelt bread pieces

One peeled, pitted, and mashed avocado

Half a cup of cherry tomatoes

Half a teaspoon of salt

two tsp key lime juice

Guidelines

1. Put the avocado in a bowl, squeeze in the lime, and mash until smooth.

2. Top each toast with an equal amount of mashed avocado, followed by cherry tomatoes.

3. Season tomatoes with salt and serve.

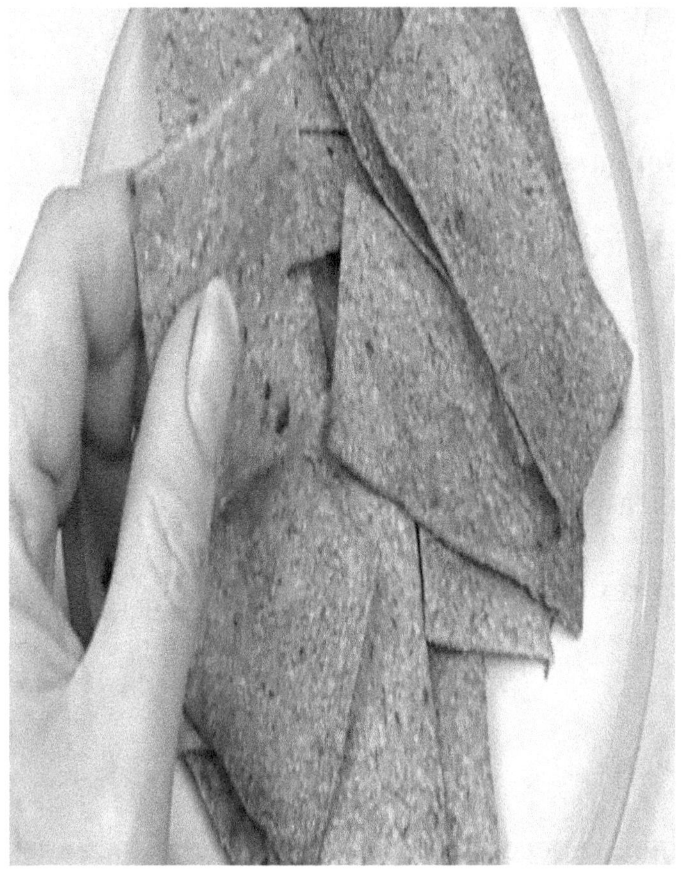

While some individuals like cakes or buns, we all know that crackers are not only incredibly appealing but also sweeping the snack industry. Who says that following Dr. Barbara's diet means you can't have crackers? a cracker with alkaline components. Have fun!

Servings: Two

Ten minutes for prep; ten minutes for cooking;

Information about nutrition: 1.2 g Fats, 0.8 g Protein, 16.4 g Carb, 1.7 g Fiber, and 81.2 Cal

Components

One cup of rye flour

One tsp powdered onion

Half a teaspoon of salt

a smidgeon of dried thyme

One-half teaspoon of dried basil

Additional: two teaspoons of grapeseed oil

Four tsp of spring water.

Guidelines

1. Turn on the oven, then warm it to 400 degrees Fahrenheit.

2. In the meantime, pulse the flour, oil, and all the spices in a food processor until well blended.

3. After adding the water and pulsing the dough until it comes together, roll it out to a thickness of ½ inch.

4. Cut out the desired shape of the cookie using a cookie cutter, place the cookies on a large baking sheet, and bake for 10 minutes, or until well browned.

5. Present immediately.

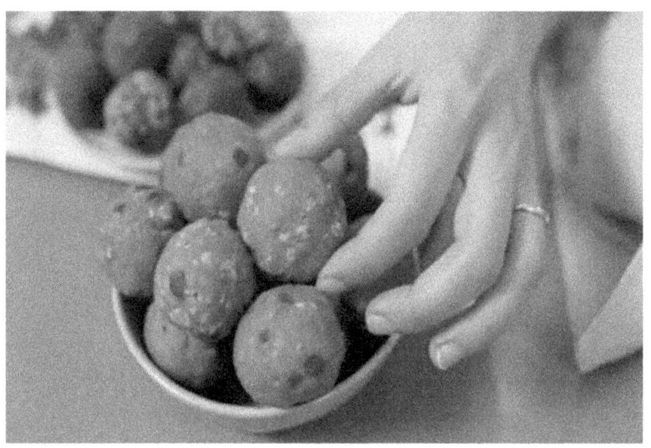

You're sure to like these calming, nutty date balls whether you're White or Black. Make it anytime you want something comforting to munch on. No eggs needed to be cracked. satisfies maybe two hungry people.

Servings: Two

Time spent preparing: five minutes; time spent cooking: none;

Information about nutrition: 5.3 g Fats, 2 g Protein, 13.5 g Carb, and 2 g Fiber; 99.1 Cal;

Components

Half a cup of walnuts

Half a cup of pitted dates

Half a cup of sesame seeds

½ cup grated soft-jelly coconut

Two tsp of agave syrup

Additional: ¼ tsp sea salt

Guidelines

1. Attach the jar to a high-speed food processor or blender, then add all ingredients except the sesame seeds.

2. Place the lid on the blender jar and pulse for 20 seconds, or until everything is well blended.

3. Transfer the mixture into a basin, form the dough into balls of uniform size, and then coat each ball with sesame seeds.

4. Serve immediately.

VEGETABLE ZOODLE SOUP

This tasty, calming soup has probably existed since Moses wandered the desert. You will adore it. When you feel very religious, make it. Eat properly and stay healthy.

Servings: Two

It takes five minutes to prepare and twelve minutes to cook.

Nutrition Facts: 265 Calories; 2 g Fats; 4 g Protein; 57 g Carb; 13.6 g Fiber;

Components

½ onion, peeled and cubed; ½ green bell pepper, diced; ½ zucchini, grated; ½ cup cherry tomatoes; 4 ounces sliced mushrooms

Bonus: ¼ cup of basil leaves

One package of cooked spelled noodles and one-half tsp salt

one-eighth teaspoon of cayenne

half a key lime squeezed

One spoonful of oil made from grapeseed

two cups of lukewarm spring water

Guidelines

1. Heat the oil in a medium saucepan over medium heat. Add the onion and cook for three minutes or until the onion is soft.

2. Stir in the bell pepper, mushrooms, and cherry tomatoes. Cook for a further three minutes, or until the ingredients are tender.

3. Include the shredded zucchini, season with the cayenne and salt, add the water, and heat the mixture until it boils.

4. After that, reduce the heat to low, stir in the cooked noodles, and boil the soup for five minutes.

5. When finished, spoon soup into two bowls, sprinkle basil leaves on top, squeeze in a little lime juice, and serve.

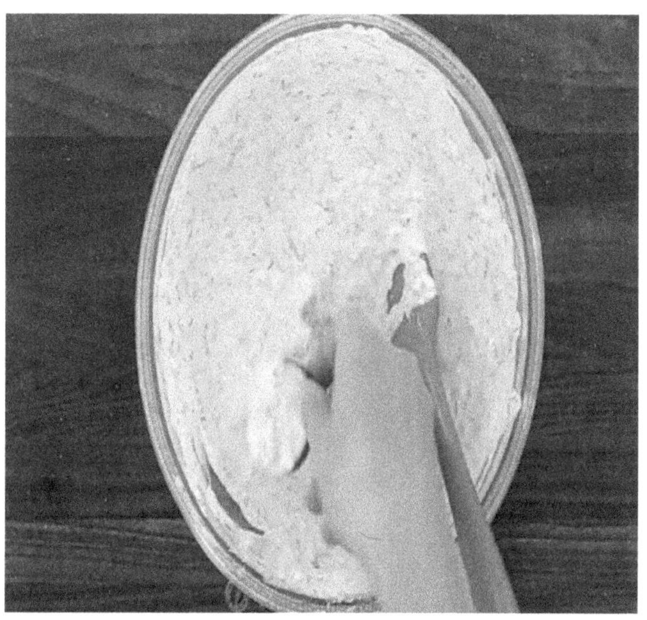

for a really hungry individual or a couple who are enjoying a lovely, romantic dinner date at their adorable small home. Your cat will adore you excessively if you don't offer her anything.

Servings: Two

Time spent preparing: five minutes; time spent cooking: none;

Information about nutrition: 15 g Fats, 4 g Protein, 15 g Carb, and 6 g Fiber; 190 Cal

Components

One chilled, peeled, pitted avocado

One cool, deseeded, peeled cucumber

½ cup cool basil leaves

half a key lime squeezed

Two cups of cool spring water

Additional: 0.5 tsp sea salt

Guidelines

1. Fill the jar in a high-speed food processor or blender with all the ingredients, and pulse to make everything smooth.

2. Transfer the soup to a medium-sized bowl and refrigerate for at least one hour.

3. Evenly divide the soup into two dishes, garnish
with more basil, and serve.

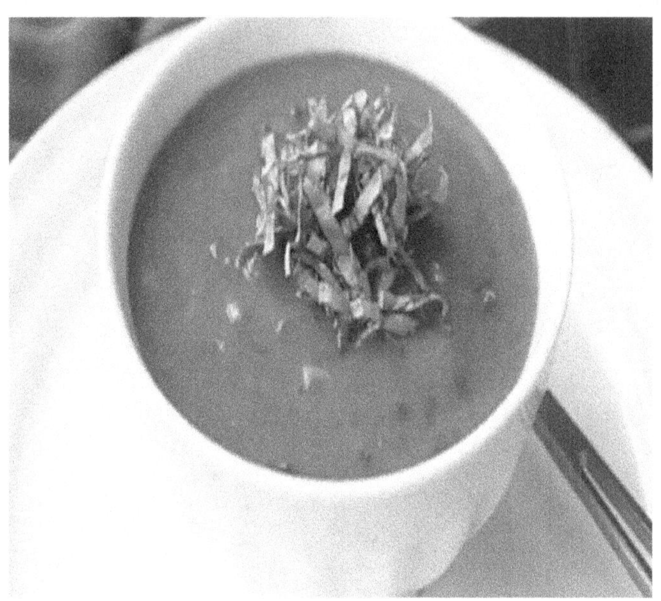

Servings: Two

Cooking time: 45 minutes; preparation time: 5 minutes.

224 calories, 5 g fats, 5.8 g protein, 38.1 g carbs, and 3.4 g fiber

Components

One cup of finely chopped kale

Two washed and torn soursop leaves cut in half

½ cup cubed summer squash

Cubed chayote squash, one cup

½ cup cubed zucchini

Bonus:

Half a cup of wild rice

Diced white onions, ½ cup

Diced green bell peppers, one cup

two tsp sea salt

½ teaspoon cayenne pepper and ½ tablespoon basil

One-third cup oregano

Six ounces of spring water

Guidelines

1. Fill a medium saucepan with 1 ½ cups water, add the soursop leaves, and cook over medium-high heat for 15 minutes while keeping the lid on.

2. After the eaves are cooked, take them from the broth, reduce the heat to medium, add the remaining ingredients, stir to combine, and simmer for an additional 30 minutes or until the food is well cooked.

3. Present immediately.

THE DELECTABLE SUN-DRIED CHICKPEA AND MUSHROOM BOWL ZUCCHINI

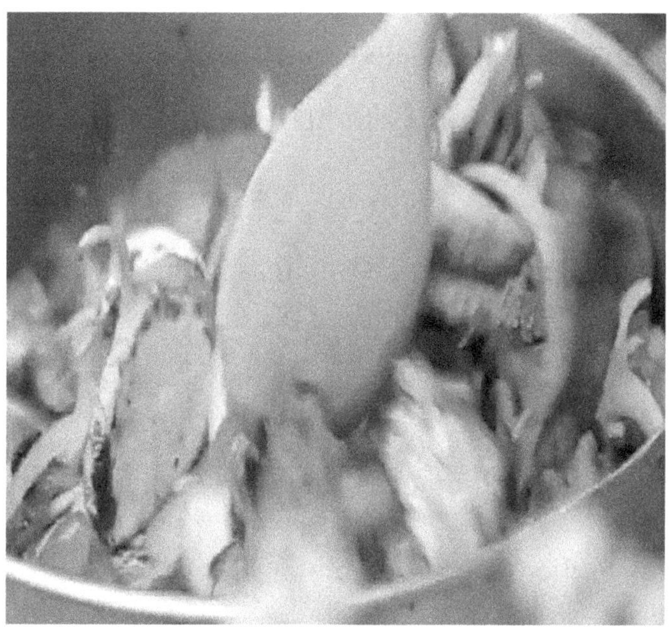

Servings: Two

It takes five minutes to prepare and ten minutes to cook.

24-2 Cal, 9 g Fats, 10 g Protein, 34 g Carb, and 9 g Fiber are the nutritional details.

Components

One-half cup of cooked chickpeas

Two spiralized zucchini

¼ of white onion, peeled and chopped; 4 tiny oyster mushrooms; ¼ of red bell pepper, cored and chopped;

Additional ingredients: ½ teaspoon cayenne pepper, ¼ teaspoon dried basil, ½ teaspoon dried oregano, and 1/3 teaspoon sea salt

One spoonful of oil made from grapeseed

2 ½ cups homemade vegetable broth

Guidelines

1. Heat the oil in a medium saucepan over medium-high heat. Add the red pepper, onion, and mushrooms. Season with salt and cayenne pepper. Cook for 5 minutes, or until the vegetables are soft.

2. Reduce the heat to medium-low, toss in the other ingredients (except the zucchini noodles), and simmer the soup for 15 to 20 minutes.

3. After that, add the zucchini noodles to the pan, swirl to combine, and cook for a further minute or so, or until they are fully heated. Serve immediately.

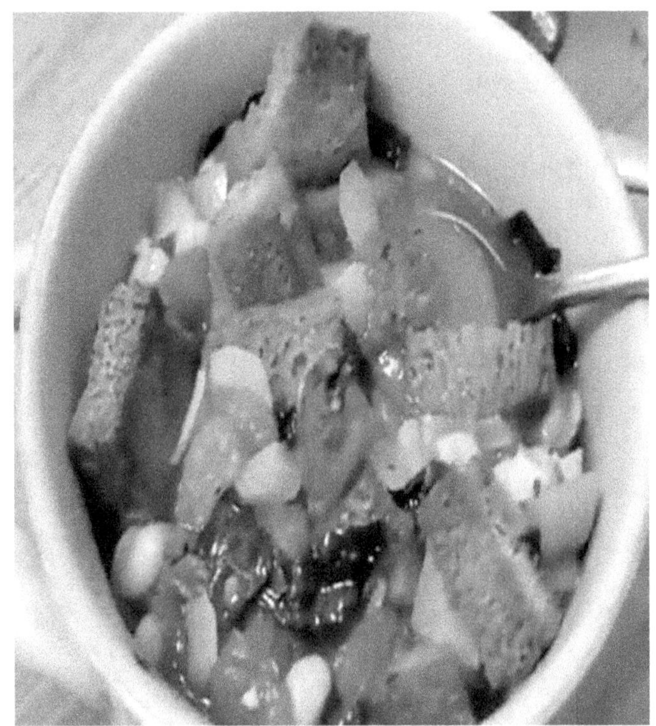

Servings: Two

It takes five minutes to prepare and twenty-five minutes to cook.

Information about nutrition: 0.3 g Fats, 6.8 g Protein, 31 g Carb, 6 g Fiber, and 184.5 Cal

Components

½ cup cooked, diced chickpeas; ½ peeled and diced medium white onion; ½ chopped big zucchini

One cup of kale leaves

One cup of cubed squash

Additives: ¾ teaspoon salt

¾ tablespoon of freshly chopped thyme

¾ tablespoon of fresh tarragon

Two cups of homemade vegetable broth

a half-cup of spring water

Guidelines

1. Fill a saucepan with 1/4 cup stock, add the onion, zucchini, and thyme, and simmer for 4 minutes over medium-high heat.

2. Add the remaining broth and water, bring to a boil, reduce heat to low, and simmer until soft, 10 to 15 minutes.

3. Add the additional ingredients, stir to combine, and simmer for a minimum of 10 minutes to ensure doneness.

4. Serve immediately.

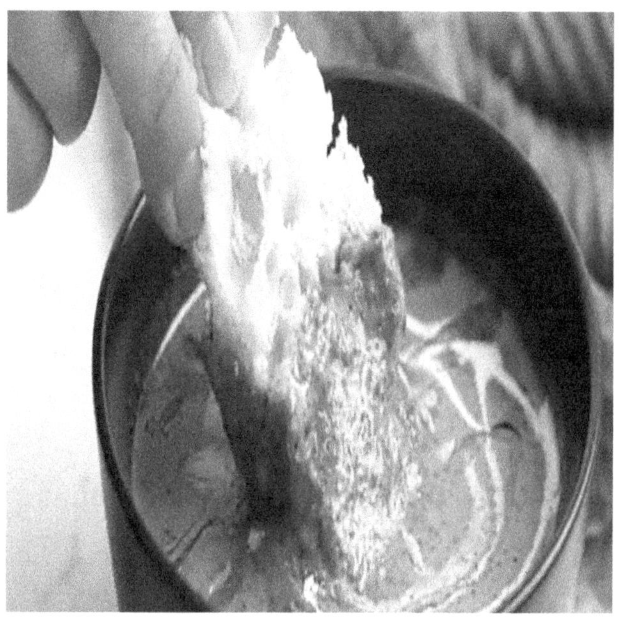

The typical soup recipe comprises a lot of seafood, but this one will replace it as fish belong in the ocean or a fish tank, not in your stomach. Have fun!

Servings: Two

Ten minutes for prep; ten minutes for cooking;

Information about nutrition: 1.2 g Fats, 1.1 g Protein, 28 g Carb, and 4.5 g Fiber; 129 Cal

Components

Two cups of leafy greens

0.5 cups of spring water; 1 small zucchini, cut; 1 small white onion, peeled and sliced; 1 medium green bell pepper, cored and sliced;

Additional: ½ teaspoon each of salt and cayenne

One tsp of dried basil

Guidelines

1. Transfer all the ingredients to a medium saucepan over medium heat, stir to combine, and simmer for 5 to 10 minutes, or until the veggies are crisp-tender.

2. Take the saucepan off of the burner, use an immersion blender to purée the soup, and serve.

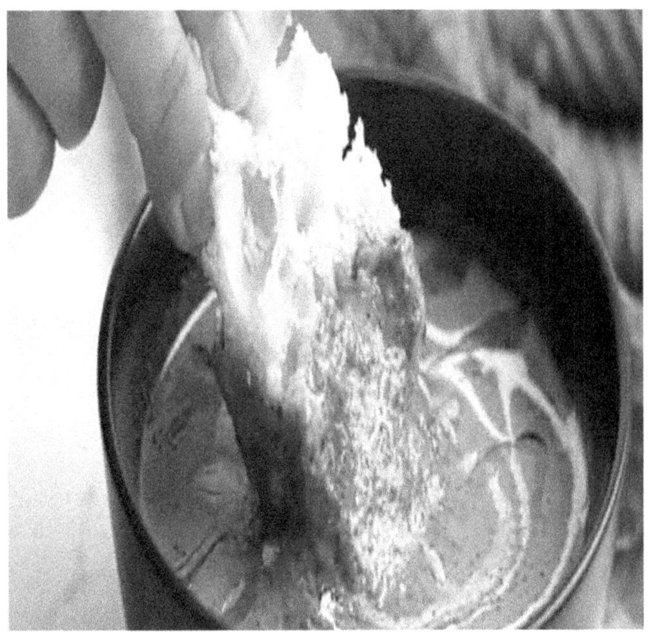

Servings: Two

5 minutes for preparation; 32 minutes for cooking;
348.8 calories; 8.8 grams of fats; 11.3 grams of
protein; 57.2 grams of carbohydrates; and 7.8
grams of fiber;

Components

Half a cup of Kamut berries

one cup of finely chopped white onion

½ cup finely sliced squash

½ cup of cooked lentils

One cup of homemade vegetable broth

Extra: half a teaspoon of cayenne

1/4 cup finely chopped tarragon

One minced thyme teaspoon and one bay leaf

One tablespoon of olive oil

One cup of boiling spring water

Guidelines

1. Transfer the Kamut to a small bowl, cover with boiling water, and leave for half an hour.

2. Next, put some oil in a medium-sized saucepan over medium heat, add the onion, whisk in the tarragon and thyme, and simmer for 5 minutes, or until the onion is soft.

3. After draining the Kamut, place it in the saucepan, add the bay leaves, cover with the vegetable broth, and heat it until it boils.

4. Place the pot's lid on top, simmer for 20 to 30 minutes, then add the cayenne pepper and let it cook for an additional five minutes.

5. Take out the bay leaf, add the chickpeas, and simmer for another two minutes.

6. Present immediately.

www.ingramcontent.com/pod-product-compliance
Lightning Source LLC
Chambersburg PA
CBHW050808250726
48653CB00006B/2151